Alkaline Appetizers & Snacks Cookbook

The Ultimate Alkaline Cookbook for Better Appetizers & Snacks

Richard Ortega

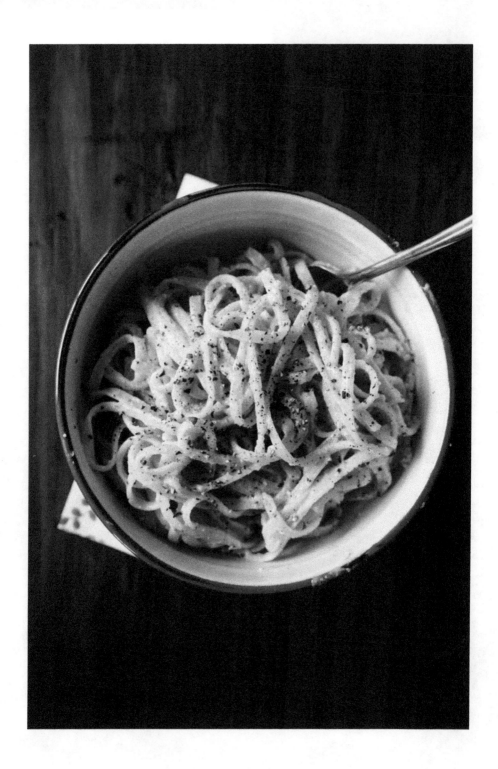

Readers acknowledge that the author is not engaging in the rendering of legal, financial, medical or professional advice. The content within this book has been derived from various sources. Please consult a licensed professional before attempting any techniques outlined in this book.

By reading this document, the reader agrees that under no circumstances is the author responsible for any losses, direct or indirect, which are incurred as a result of the use of information contained within this document, including, but not limited to, — errors, omissions, or inaccuracies.

TABLE OF CONTENTS

Avocado Basil Pasta

Preparation Time: 10 minutes

Cooking Time: 15 minutes

Servings: 4

Ingredients:

- 4 cups Cooked spelt pasta
- ¼ cup Olive oil
- 1 tsp Agave syrup
- 1 tbsp Key lime juice
- 1-pint Halved cherry tomatoes
- 1 cup Chopped basil
- 1 Chopped avocado

Directions:

1. In a bowl, put in the cooked pasta then mix in the tomatoes, basil, and avocado. Toss to combine.
2. Put the salt, agave syrup, lime juice, and oil into a bowl. You are going to need to whisk everything vigorously in order to get everything combined. Pour dressing on top of the pasta mixture. Now toss everything together to coat the pasta with the dressing.

Nutrition:

254 calories | 8g fat 7g protein

Kale and Brazil Nut Pesto with Butternut Squash

Preparation Time: 15 minutes

Cooking Time: 20 minutes

Servings: 3

Ingredients:

- Squash:
- Sea salt
- 1 tbsp Dried sage
- 1 tbsp Grapeseed oil
- 1 ½ cup Cubed butternut squash
- Pesto:
- 2 tsp Onion powder.
- 2 tbsp Chopped Brazil nuts
- 4 tbsp Olive oil
- Juice of 2 limes
- 1 tbsp Parsley
- 2 cups Kale
- 2 ½ cup Cooked quinoa

Directions:

1. To start, get your oven to 400. Add the butternut squash to a bowl and drizzle in the oil. Add in the seasonings and toss everything to squash well. Pour the squash onto a baking sheet and allow it to bake for at least 30 minutes. Once it can be pierced easily with a fork, it is finished.

2. As the squash is cooking, add the kale, parsley, lime juice, olive oil, brazil nuts, and onion powder to your food processor. Turn the processor on and allow everything to mix together until it all comes together. The pesto may appear dry, but that's okay. This process may be loud because of the nuts.

3. Next, place cooked quinoa in a glass bowl and add in the pesto you just made. Mix them together until the pesto is evenly distributed throughout the quinoa. Add in the cooked butternut squash and toss everything together. Garnish this with a wedge of avocado and some basil. Enjoy.

Nutrition:

304 calories | 10g protein | 16g fat

Zoodles in Avocado Sauce

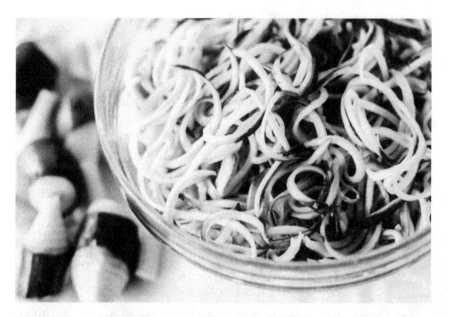

Preparation Time: 10 minutes

Cooking Time: 25 minutes

Servings: 6

Ingredients:

- Sea salt, to taste
- 24 Cherry tomatoes, sliced
- 2 Avocados
- 4 tbsp Key lime juice
- ½ cup Walnuts
- ½ cup Water
- 2 cups Basil

- 2 large Zucchinis

Directions:

1. You will need to make the zoodles by either using a spiralizer or a peeler. Place salt, avocados, lime juice, walnuts, and basil into a blender and process until creamy.
2. Place the zoodles into a bowl. Add tomatoes, avocado sauce, and zoodles. Toss until well coated. Enjoy.

Nutrition:

189 calories | 18g fiber | 24g protein

Fried Rice

Preparation Time: 10 minutes

Cooking Time: 20 minutes

Servings: 6

Ingredients:

- Cayenne pepper, to taste
- Sea salt to taste
- 1 tbsp Grapeseed oil
- ¼ cup Diced onion
- ½ cup Sliced zucchini
- ½ cup Sliced mushrooms
- ½ cup Sliced bell peppers
- 1 cup Cooked quinoa or wild rice

Directions:

1. Place a skillet on top of stove and warm grapeseed oil. Add onion and cook until slightly browned and softened.
2. To the skillet, put all the other veggies and cook these for five more minutes. They should be soft but not mushy. Add rice, stir to combine, and cook until slightly browned.

Nutrition:

129 calories | 15g fiber | 12g protein

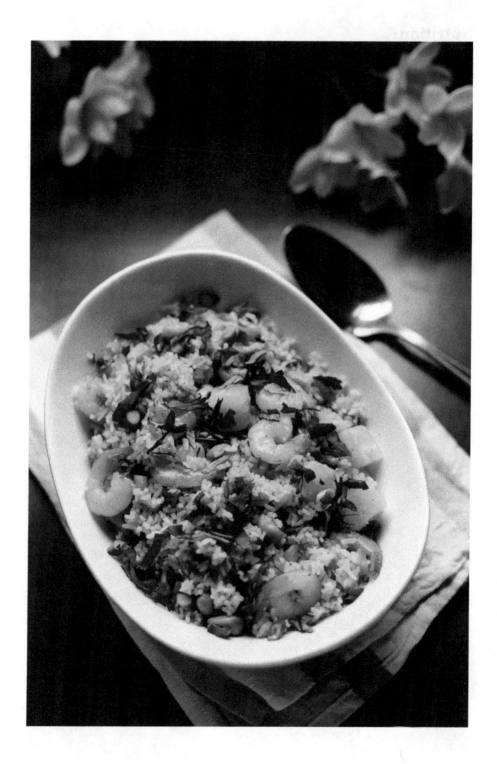

Rice and Spinach Balls

Preparation Time: 10 minutes

Cooking Time: 20 minutes

Servings: 10

Ingredients:

- For Part One
- Juice of one key lime
- 1/3 cup Pitted Greek olives
- ¾ tsp Sea salt
- 4 ½ cup Spinach leaves
- 1 tsp Onion powder
- For Part Two
- ½ cup Chickpea flour
- ½ cup Ground almonds
- 1 ¼ cup Cooked wild rice

Directions:

1. Warm your oven to 360. Place all the ingredients for part one into either a food processor or a blender whichever one you have access to. Turn on the device until everything is well combined.

2. Add this mixture to a large bowl and add in all the ingredients for part two. Combine it together to

create a dough. Mix in some flour, if the mixture seems to be too wet. You can add in some cayenne pepper for taste if you would like. I don't recommend that you taste this as chickpea flour can be very bitter.

3. Take this mixture and scoop it out with a spoon. Roll it until it turns into a ball. Place these onto a cookie sheet that has parchment paper on it. This should make one dozen balls. Place into the oven for 20 minutes. If you want to check for doneness, you will have to taste one of them. Be careful not to burn your mouth. If you don't taste any bitterness, they are done.

Nutrition:

159 calories | 14g protein | 5g fats

Flatbread

Preparation Time: 10 minutes

Cooking Time: 15 minutes

Servings: 6

Ingredients:

- 1 tbsp Sea salt
- ¼ tsp Cayenne
- 2 tsp Oregano.
- ¾ cup Springwater
- 2 tsp Onion powder
- 2 tbsp Grapeseed oil
- 2 tsp Basil, 2 tsp.

Directions:

1. Combine the seasonings together into the flour. Stir in the oil, and mix in a half cup of the water.
2. Slowly add in the rest of the water until the dough forms a ball.
3. Sprinkle some flour over your workspace and then knead your dough for five minutes. Divide it into six parts.
4. Roll the balls into four-inch circles.

5. Lay them out on an ungreased skillet that has been heated to medium-high. Flip it every two to three minutes, or until it is cooked through. Enjoy.

Nutrition:

180 calories | 18g protein | 10g fats

Chickpea "Tuna" Salad

Preparation Time: 10 minutes

Cooking Time: 20 minutes

Servings: 4

Ingredients:

- ¼ tsp Sea salt
- 1 tsp Dill
- 2 tsp Onion powder
- ½ Nori sheet
- ¼ cup Diced red onions
- 2/3 cup Alkaline mayo
- 1/8 cup Diced green peppers
- 2 cup Cooked chickpeas

Directions:

1. Crush the chickpeas in a bowl until they reached your desired consistency.
2. Slice the nori sheets up and mix them into the chickpeas. Add in all of the other ingredients and stir them together. Place the salad into the fridge for 30 minutes to an hour before you serve.

Nutrition:

200 calories | 19g protein | 5g sugar

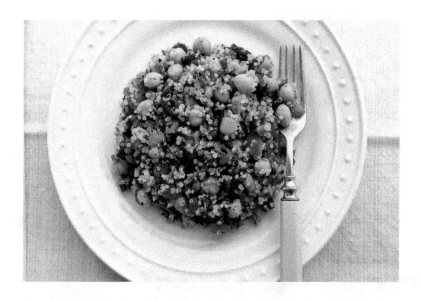

Enoki Mushroom Pasta

Preparation Time: 15 minutes

Cooking Time: 20 minutes

Servings: 4

Ingredients:

- Sea salt
- 1 tbsp Coconut oil
- Onions
- Bell pepper
- Handful of plum tomatoes
- 10.5oz Enoki mushrooms
- 2 round slices Butternut squash

Directions:

1. Start by getting your butternut squash ready. Remove the skin of the squash then dice them up. Place the squash into a pot and let it begin boiling, cooking until soft. Once they are soft, pour out the water and then mash then into a paste.
2. Juice your tomatoes and then mix this into your squash. This will thin the squash paste out a bit and will add more flavor. You can add in some Irish moss jelly at this point, but you don't have to.

3. Mix in the onion, bell pepper, and mushrooms. Allow this all to simmer together for two to five minutes.

4. Then add in some salt to taste. Allow this to cool for five to ten minutes and then stir in the coconut oil. The coconut oil will create a really nice rich flavor. Enjoy.

Nutrition:

150 calories | 12g fiber | 5g sugar

Pasta with Walnut Pesto

Preparation Time: 10 minutes

Cooking Time: 25 minutes

Servings: 4

Ingredients:

- ½ cup Walnuts
- Juice of a lime
- Sea salt
- 3 cup Fresh basil
- Avocado
- ½ cup Spelt pasta

Directions:

1. To start, add the basil, avocado, walnuts, lime juice, and salt to a food processor. Blend well all the ingredients to form a smooth sauce.

2. Next, cook your spelt pasta according to the directions on the packaging. Once cooked, drain, and pour into a bowl. Pour in the pesto and mix everything together. At this point, you can mix in some extra Alkaline approved ingredients like chopped olives, chopped tomatoes, and torn basil. Enjoy.

Nutrition:

190 calories | 4g sugar | 18g fat

Walnut Kale Pasta

Preparation Time: 12 minutes

Cooking Time: 20 minutes

Servings: 6

Ingredients:

- Cayenne pepper to taste
- Sea salt to taste
- 2 tbsp Avocado oil
- 1 small Chopped onion
- 1/3 cup Walnut flakes
- 1 ½ cup Spelt pasta
- 3 cups Kale

Directions:

1. Begin by fixing the pasta the way the package tells you to. It still needs to be "al dente."
2. Wash the kale and chop into bite-size pieces.
3. Put the avocado oil in a large skillet and slowly heat it up then add the onion. Allow the onion to cook until it has softened and turned a translucent color now put the kale into the skillet and stir to combine with onions. Add some water and cook until kale is wilted.

4. In another dry skillet, add the walnut flakes and toast gently.

5. Once the kale is wilted, add pasta, and stir well to combine.

6. Sprinkle with walnut flakes and season to taste.

Nutrition:

204 calories | 18g protein | 5g sugar

Tomato Pasta

Preparation Time: 15 minutes

Cooking Time: 20 minutes

Servings: 4

Ingredients:

- 1lb Spelt pasta
- 2 tbsp Olive oil
- 1 Bell pepper
- 1 medium Zucchini
- 1 large Onion
- 1 (15 oz) can Chickpeas
- 5 Chopped tomatoes

Directions:

1. Start by fixing the pasta the way the package tells you to.
2. Wash and chop the zucchini, onion, bell pepper, and tomatoes. Add to a skillet along with some water.
3. "Steam fry" the vegetables until tender.
4. Drain and rinse the chickpeas. Put them in the tomato mixture and cook five minutes or until they have been warmed through.

5. Drain the pasta and divide it evenly into plates. Divide the sauce evenly and pour on the pasta. If you want the extra flavor, you can drizzle some olive oil on top and enjoy.

Nutrition:

116 calories | 9g fat | 13g protein

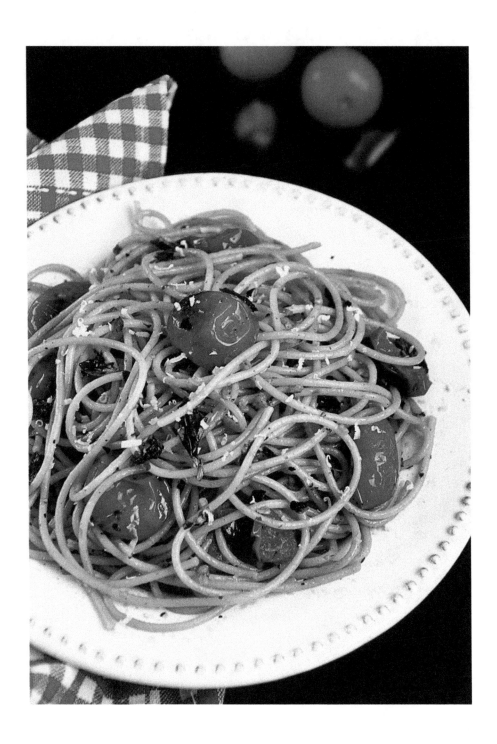

Spicy Sesame Ginger Noodle Bowl

Preparation Time: 10 minutes

Cooking Time: 20 minutes

Servings: 6

Ingredients:

- 8 oz Spelt angel hair pasta
- 2 tbsp Sesame oil
- 1 Peeled and chopped cucumber
- 1 tsp Onion powder
- 1 tbsp Walnut butter
- 1 tbsp Tahini
- Juice of one key lime
- 1 tbsp Grated ginger
- Sea salt to taste
- Cayenne pepper to taste

Directions:

1. Fix the pasta as per the directions on the package. Drain and rinse with cool water. Leave in colander while you make the dressing.

2. Add the onion powder, ginger, lime juice, sesame oil, tahini, walnut butter, cayenne, salt, and cucumber to a small bowl. Whisk until walnut butter and tahini are incorporated together. Taste and adjust seasonings if needed.

3. Transfer the pasta in a large bowl then drizzle dressing over the top. Toss to coat.

4. You may garnish with black sesame seeds and lime wedges if desired.

Nutrition:

130 calories | 15g fiber | 20g protein

Zucchini Tomato Pasta

Preparation Time: 10 minutes

Cooking Time: 25 minutes

Servings: 4

Ingredients:

- 2 Key lime wedges,
- 2 medium Zucchinis
- Sea salt to taste
- 1 tsp Basil
- 2 Chopped tomatoes
- 1 tsp Oregano
- 1 medium Chopped onion
- 2 tsp Avocado oil

Directions:

1. Begin by warming some avocado oil in a skillet. Add the onion to the skillet and let the onion cook until it has softened. Add in salt, oregano, basil, and tomatoes. Stir well and continue cooking until the tomatoes are soft and the ingredients have cooked together. This will take about four minutes.

2. Using either a spiralizer or peeled, turn the zucchini into noodles. Divide them equally between two plates. Add one lime wedge to each plate.

3. If you want your zucchini heated through, you can add it to the sauce for a minute. Cooking the zucchini for too long will lose some of its nutrients.

4. When ready to eat, squeeze the lime over the pasta and enjoy.

Nutrition:

150 calories | 17g protein | 9g fiber

Creamy Mushroom Pasta

Preparation Time: 15 minutes

Cooking Time: 30 minutes

Servings: 6

Ingredients:

- Cayenne pepper to taste
- 3 cups Coconut milk
- Sea salt to taste
- 3 tbsp Chickpea Flour
- 8 cups Mixed mushrooms
- 1 medium Chopped onion
- ¼ cup Avocado oil
- 1lb. Spelt pasta

Directions:

1. In a large pasta pot, pour eight cups water and add a large handful of sea salt. Cook the pasta like the package states. When done, drain.
2. While the pasta cooks, you can get the sauce ready.
3. Warm the avocado oil in a skillet. Place the onions, mushroom, and a pinch of salt. Cook while occasionally stirring until mushrooms have softened and are slightly browned. This will take about 15

minutes. Turn the heat down after five minutes have passed.

4. Sprinkle the flour over the mushroom mixture and stir well. Make sure everything is covered with the flour. Let this cook for about one minute. Turn the heat back on.

5. Add in one cup of the coconut milk while constantly stirring and simmer for one minute. Break up any clumps that might have formed.

6. Once it is totally smooth and has thickened a bit, add the rest of the coconut milk. Add some cayenne for your taste and bring the liquid to a simmer while constantly stirring.

7. Continue cooking until the sauce has thickened one more time.

8. Take off heat. Taste and adjust seasonings if needed.

9. Place the cooked pasta into the sauce. Toss well to coat everything.

10. Divide into serving plates and enjoy.

Nutrition:

160 calories | 18g fiber | 24g protein

Zucchini Burritos

Preparation Time: 15 minutes

Cooking Time: 25 minutes

Servings: 4

Ingredients:

- Sesame seeds
- 1 tbsp Tahini
- Sprouted hemp seeds handful
- Dandelion greens or amaranth handful
- 1 small Zucchini, cut into rounds
- 4 sheets Nori seaweed
- ½ Sliced mango
- Cucumber
- Sliced avocado

Directions:

1. Put the Nori sheets onto a cutting board. Make sure the shiny side is facing the cutting board.
2. Place all the ingredients onto the Nori in whatever arrangement you would like. Leave about one inch uncovered on the right side of the Nori.
3. Use both hands and begin folding the Nori from the side closest to you. Roll it over the filling.

4. Slice into two-inch thick slices and sprinkle over sesame seeds.

Nutrition:

118 calories | 5g fats | 13g protein

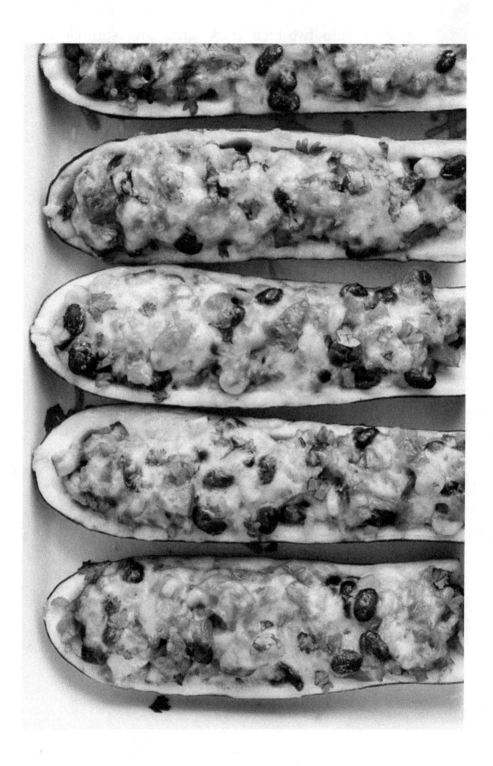

Zucchini Bacon

Preparation Time: 10 minutes

Cooking Time: 6 minutes

Servings: 4

Ingredients:

- 3 zucchinis, sliced thinly lengthwise or into large strips
- 1/4 cup date sugar
- 1/4 cup spring water
- 1 tablespoon sea salt
- 1 tablespoon onion powder
- 1/2 teaspoon cayenne pepper powder
- 1/2 teaspoon ground ginger
- 1 tablespoon liquid smoke
- Grapeseed oil for frying

Directions:

1. Except for the grapeseed, put all the ingredients in a bowl.
2. Allow the zucchini strips to marinate for at least 2 hours in the fridge.
3. On the Instant Pot, press the Sauté button and heat the oil until it slightly smokes.

4. Fry the marinated zucchini strips for 3 minutes on each side until crispy.

Nutrition:

36 Calories | 0.64g Protein | 8.7g Carbs | 6.5g Sugar | 0.09g Fat

Alkaline Spelt Bread

Preparation Time: 15 minutes

Cooking Time: 6 hours

Servings: 8

Ingredients:

- 4-1/2 cups spelt flour
- 2 teaspoons sea salt
- 2 cups spring water
- 1/4 cup agave
- Grapeseed oil for brushing the bread
- A dash of sesame seeds

Directions:

1. In mixing the ingredients use hook attachment of the mixer.
2. Sift together the spelt flour and salt in a bowl. Place in a mixer and mix for 10 seconds.
3. Add in the water and agave. Mix for 10 minutes until the dough is formed.
4. Coat the dough with grapeseed oil and place in a clean bowl. Let it rest for at least 1 hour.
5. At the bottom of the Instant Pot, line it with parchment paper.

6. Sprinkle the dough with sesame seeds and place inside the Instant Pot.

7. Close the lid but do not set the vent to the Sealing position.

8. Press the Slow Cook button and adjust the cooking time to 6 hours.

Nutrition:

331 Calories | 14.3g Protein | 68.7g Carbs | 6.7g Sugar | 2.4g Fat

Alkaline Crustless Quiche

Preparation Time: 15 minutes

Cooking Time: 4 hours

Servings: 4

Ingredients:

- 1 cup garbanzos bean flour
- 3/4 cup fresh coconut milk
- 1 tablespoon sea salt
- 1 tablespoon oregano
- 1/4 teaspoon cayenne pepper
- 2 cups mushrooms, sliced
- 1 cup kale, chopped
- 1/2 cup white onions, chopped
- 1/2 cup yellow peppers, seeded and chopped

Directions:

1. Place the garbanzos bean flour, coconut milk, salt, oregano, and cayenne pepper. Mix until a smooth batter is formed.
2. Stir in the rest of the ingredients.
3. Place a parchment paper in the bottom of the Instant Pot and pour over the mixture.

4. Close the lid but do not set the vent to the Sealing position.

5. Press the Slow Cook button and adjust the cooking time to 4 hours.

Nutrition:

328 Calories | 12.1g Protein | 40g Carbs | 7.3g Sugar | 14.9g Fat

Alkaline's Home Fries Hash browns

Preparation Time: 15 minutes

Cooking Time: 6 minutes

Servings: 6

Ingredients:

- 3 green bananas, peeled and chopped
- 1/4 cup onion
- 1/4 cup green pepper
- 1 plum tomato, diced
- 1 teaspoon sea salt
- 1 teaspoon oregano
- 1/2 teaspoon cayenne powder
- Grapeseed oil for frying

Directions:

1. Except for the grapeseed oil, put all the ingredients in a bowl. Mix until well-combined.
2. Press the Sauté button on the Instant Pot and heat the oil.
3. Get a tablespoon of the mixture and place in the Instant Pot. Flatten to form a small pancake.

4. Cook for 3 minutes on all sides.

5. Do the same thing to the rest of the mixture.

Nutrition: 77 Calories | 0.66g Protein | 13.4g Carbs | 7.8g Sugar | 3g Fat

Alkaline Blueberry and Strawberry Muffins

Preparation Time: 15 minutes

Cooking Time: 5 hours

Servings: 6

Ingredients:

- 3/4 cup quinoa flour
- 3/4 cup teff flour
- 1/2 teaspoon salt
- 1/3 cup agave
- 1 cup fresh coconut milk
- 1/4 cup strawberries, chopped
- 1/4 cup blueberries

Directions:

1. Place the quinoa flour, teff flour, and salt in a bowl.
2. In another bowl, combine the agave and coconut milk. Slowly pour the wet ingredients to the dry ingredients. Mix until well-combined. Stir in the berries and mix until well-combined.
3. Pour the batter in muffin pans. Place the muffin pans with the batter in the Instant Pot.

4. Close the lid but do not set the vent to the Sealing position.

5. Press the Slow Cook button and adjust the cooking time to 4 to 5 hours.

Nutrition:

271 Calories | 7.2g Protein | 36.6g Carbs | 4.3g Sugar | 11.5g Fat

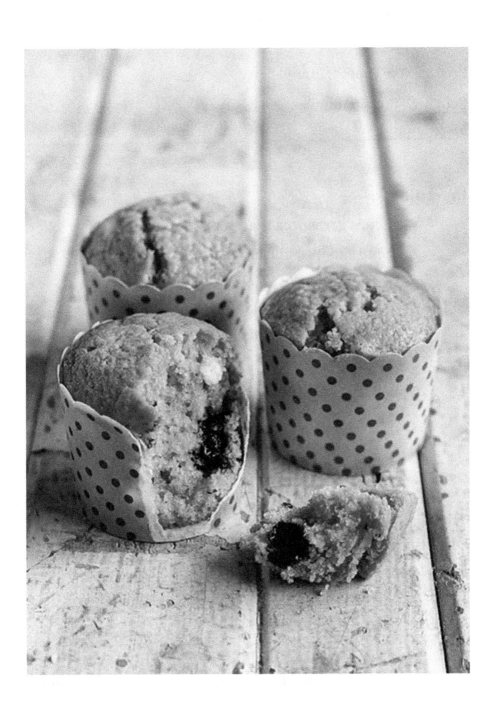

Alkaline Sausage Links

Preparation Time: 15 minutes

Cooking Time: 6 minutes

Servings: 6

Ingredients:

- 2 cups garbanzos beans flour
- 1 cup chopped mushrooms
- 1/2 cup chopped onions
- 1 tomato, chopped
- 1 teaspoon oregano
- 1 teaspoon sea salt
- 1 teaspoon ground sage
- 1 teaspoon dill, chopped
- 1/2 teaspoon cayenne pepper powder
- Grapeseed oil for frying

Directions:

1. Except for the grapeseed oil, put all the ingredients in a bowl. Combine all the ingredients with your hands. Create small logs of sausages and place inside the fridge to set for at least 30 minutes.
2. Pour oil in the Instant Pot and press the Sauté button until the oil is hot.

3. Place the sausage links carefully and cook on all sides for 3 minutes.

Nutrition:

266 Calories | 14.6g Protein | 44.9g Carbs | 8.6g Sugar | 4.2g Fat

Butternut Squash Hash Browns

Preparation Time: 15 minutes

Cooking Time: 6 minutes

Servings: 3

Ingredients:

- 1/2 cup butternut squash
- 1/2 cup diced onion
- A dash of sea salt
- A dash of cayenne pepper powder
- Grapeseed oil for brushing the Instant Pot

Directions:

1. Shred the butternut squash and place in a bowl. Add the onion, salt, and cayenne pepper.
2. Mix until well-combined. Create small patties using the mixture. Pour grapeseed oil in the Instant Pot and press the Sauté button.
3. Place the hash brown in the Instant Pot and cook for 3 minutes on all sides.

Nutrition:

64 Calories | 0.7g Protein | 5.9g Carbs | 2.1g Sugar | 4.6g Fat

Blueberry Spelt Flat Cakes

Preparation Time: 15 minutes

Cooking Time: 4 hours

Servings: 4

Ingredients:

- 2 cups spelt flour
- 1/4 teaspoon sea salt
- 1/4 cup hemp seeds
- 1 cup fresh coconut milk
- 1/2 cup spring water
- 2 tablespoons grapeseed oil
- 1/2 cup agave
- 1/2 cup blueberries

Directions:

1. In a bowl, mix the spelt flour, sea salt, and hemp seeds. Pour in the coconut milk, water, grapeseed oil, and agave. Stir until well-combined. Pour in the blueberries.
2. Line the Instant Pot with parchment paper. Pour the batter into the Instant Pot. Close the lid but do not set the vent to the Sealing position.

3. Press the Slow Cook button and adjust the cooking time to 4 hours.

Nutrition:

574 Calories | 16.1g Protein | 74.8g Carbs | 14.8g Sugar | 27.8g Fat

Garlicky Broccoli

Preparation Time: 10 minutes

Cooking Time: 8 minutes

Servings: 2

Ingredients:

- 1 tablespoon olive oil
- 2 garlic cloves, minced
- 2 cups broccoli florets
- 2 tablespoons water
- salt and black pepper to taste

Directions:

1. Cook the oil over medium heat in a skillet and sauté the garlic for about 1 minute.
2. Add the broccoli and stir fry for 2 minutes.
3. Stir in water, salt, and black pepper and stir fry for 4-5 minutes.
4. Serve hot.

Nutrition:

95 Calories | 7.3g Total Fat | 148 mg Sodium | 7g Total Carbs | 2.4g Fiber

Sautéed Kale

Preparation Time: 10 minutes

Cooking Time: 20 minutes

Servings: 4

Ingredients:

- 1 tablespoon extra-virgin olive oil
- 1 lemon, seeded and sliced thinly
- 1 onion, sliced thinly
- 3 garlic cloves, minced
- 2 pounds fresh kale, trimmed and chopped
- ½ cup scallions, chopped
- salt and black pepper to taste

Directions:

1. Cook the oil over medium heat in a skillet and cook the lemon slices for 5 minutes.
2. With a slotted spoon, remove the lemon slices from skillet and set aside.
3. In the same skillet, add the onion and garlic and sauté for about 5 minutes.
4. Add the kale, scallions, honey, salt, and pepper and cook for 8-10 minutes.

5. Add the lemon slices and mix until well combined. Serve hot.

Nutrition: 161 Calories | 3.6g Total Fat | 28.3g Total Carbs | 4.6g Fiber | 1.6g Sugar | 7.5g Protein

Parsley Mushrooms

Preparation Time: 15 minutes

Cooking Time: 14 minutes

Servings: 2

Ingredients:

- 2 tablespoons olive oil
- 2-3 tablespoons onion, minced
- ½ teaspoon garlic, minced
- 12 ounces fresh mushrooms, sliced
- 1 tablespoon fresh parsley
- salt and black pepper to taste

Directions:

1. Cook the oil over medium heat in a skillet and sauté the onion and garlic for 2-3 minutes.
2. Add the mushrooms and cook for 8-10 minutes or until desired doneness.
3. Stir in the parsley salt and black pepper and remove from the heat.
4. Serve hot.

Nutrition:

162 Calories | 14.5g Total Fat | 6.9g Total Carbs | 2g Fiber | 3.4g Sugar

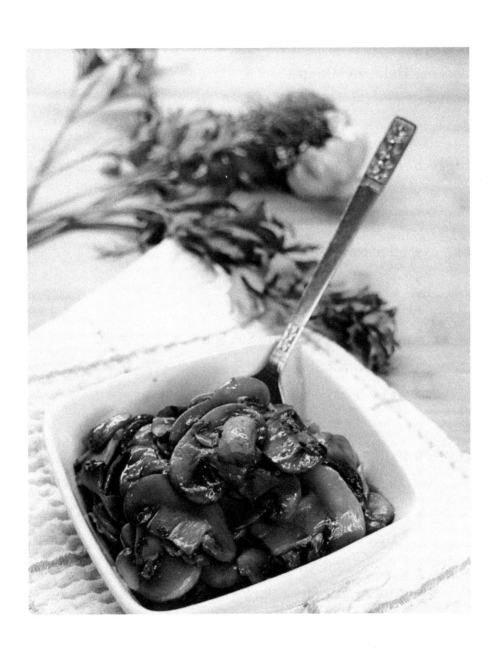

Speltbread

Preparation Time: 10 minutes

Cooking Time: 20 Minutes

Servings: 6

Ingredients:

- 2 cups of Spelt Flour
- 2 teaspoons of Oregano
- 2 teaspoons of Onion Powder
- 1/4 teaspoon of Cayenne
- 2 teaspoons of Basil
- 1 tablespoon of Pure Sea Salt
- 3/4 cup of Spring Water
- 2 tablespoons of Grape Seed Oil

Directions:

1. Add the Spelt Flour and all seasonings into a medium bowl and mix them well. Add the Grape Seed Oil and 1/2 cup of Spring Water and continue to mix.
2. Try to form the mixture into a dough ball. If it is too thick, add more Spring Water. Prepare a place for rolling out the dough and cover it with flour.

3. Knead the dough for about 5 minutes until it achieves the desired consistency. Divide the dough into 6 equal balls.

4. Roll out each ball into circles about 4 inches in diameter. Heat a non-stick pan. Transfer one flatbread and heat it in a pan on medium heat.

5. Flip the Flatbread every 2 to 3 minutes and cook until it is done. Small golden-brown spots should appear on both sides. Continue to cook the rest of the pieces.

Nutrition:

287 Calories | 29.5g Fat | 5.9g Carbs | 4.2g Protein | 4.3g Fiber

Tortillas

Preparation Time: 10 minutes

Cooking Time: 20 Minutes

Servings: 8

Ingredients:

- 2 cups of Spelt Flour
- 1 teaspoon of Pure Sea Salt
- 1/2 cup of Spring Water

Directions:

1. Combine the Spelt Flour with Pure Sea Salt in a food processor*. Mix for about 15 seconds.
2. Continue blending, slowly add Grape Seed Oil until well incorporated.
3. Slowly add Spring Water while blending until a dough is formed. Cover your work surface with parchment paper. Sprinkle with flour.
4. Knead the dough until it achieves the right consistency.
5. Divide the dough into 8 equal balls.
6. Roll out each ball into a very thin circle.

7. Heat a non-stick pan, cook one tortilla at a time on medium heat for about 30 to 60 seconds on each side.

Nutrition:

248 Calories | 15.7g Fat | 0.4g Carbs | 24.9g Protein

Tortilla Chips

Preparation Time: 10 minutes

Cooking Time: 30 Minutes

Servings: 8

Ingredients:

- 2 cups of Spelt Flour
- 1 teaspoon of Pure Sea Salt
- 1/2 cup of Spring Water
- 1/3 cup of Grape Seed Oil

Directions:

1. Preheat your oven to 350 degrees Fahrenheit.
2. Combine the Spelt Flour with Pure Sea Salt in a food processor*. Mix for about 15 seconds.
3. While blending, slowly add Grape Seed Oil until it is well combined.
4. Continue to blend and slowly add Spring Water until a dough is formed.
5. Cover your work surface with parchment paper. Sprinkle flour over the paper.
6. Knead the dough until it achieves the right consistency.
7. Cover a baking pan with a little Grape Seed Oil.

8. Put the prepared dough on the baking pan.

9. Brush dough with a little Grape Seed Oil and sprinkle with more Pure Sea Salt if desired.

10. Slice the dough into 8 triangles.

11. Bake until the chips are starting to become golden brown.

12. Allow to cool before serving.

Nutrition:

80 Calories | 3.5g Fat | 11.6g Carbs | 1.2g Protein | 0.7g Fiber

Onion Rings

Preparation Time: 10 minutes

Cooking Time: 30 Minutes

Servings: 8

Ingredients:

- White Onions or Sweet Onions
- 1 cup of Spelt Flour
- 1/2 cup of Homemade Hempseed Milk
- 1/2 cup of Aquafaba
- 2 teaspoons of Onion Powder
- 2 teaspoons of Oregano
- 1 teaspoon of Cayenne Powder
- 2 teaspoons of Pure Sea Salt
- 3 tablespoons of Grape Seed Oil

Directions:

1. Preheat your oven to 450 degrees Fahrenheit.
2. Pour Homemade Hempseed Milk and Aquafaba into a medium bowl and whisk them well.
3. Mix in 1 teaspoon of oregano, 1 teaspoon of onion powder, ½ teaspoon of cayenne, and 1 teaspoon of pure sea salt to the wet ingredients and mix.
4. Peel the Onions, slice off the ends.

5. Cut the peeled onion into slices about 1/4 inch thick. Separate the onion slices into rings.

6. Add Spelt Flour, 1 teaspoon of Oregano, 1 teaspoon of Onion Powder, 1/2 teaspoon of Cayenne, and 1 teaspoon of Pure Sea Salt to a container with a lid. Shake all the dry ingredients well.

7. Brush a baking sheet with Grape Seed Oil

8. Place a few onion rings in the wet mixture.

9. Put wet onion rings in the dry mixture and flip until coated on both sides Put the covered onion rings on the baking sheet. Repeat steps 8 through 10 until all onion rings are covered.

10. Lightly drizzle the rings with Grape Seed Oil. Bake for about 10 to 15 minutes until golden brown.

Nutrition:

153 Calories | 7.5g Fat | 20.4g Carbs | 3.1g Protein

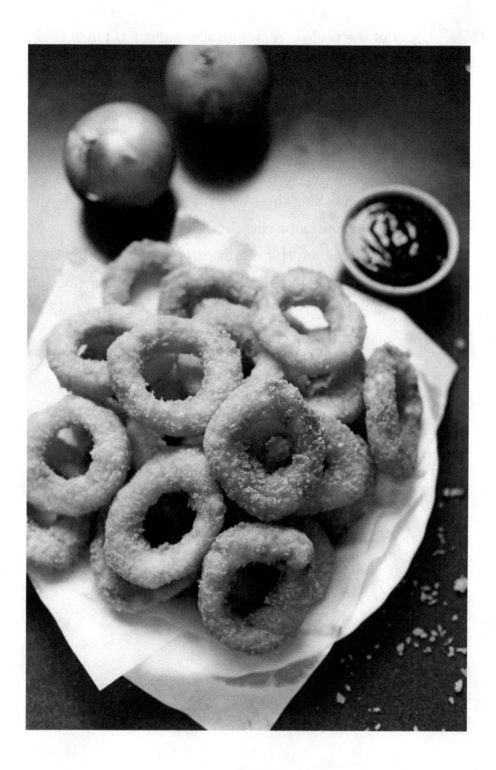

Basil and Olive Pizza

Preparation Time: 10 minutes

Cooking Time: 30 minutes

Serving: 4

Ingredients

- For the pizza sauce
- 1 (15-ounce) can tomatoes
- 1 tablespoon extra-virgin olive oil
- ½ cup fresh basil leaves, rinsed
- 2 garlic cloves, chopped
- 1 teaspoon onion powder
- ¼ teaspoon dried oregano
- ¼ teaspoon dried sage
- ¼ teaspoon dried rosemary
- ¼ teaspoon red chili flakes (optional)
- 1 teaspoon Himalayan pink salt
- Pinch freshly ground black pepper
- For the pizzas
- 4 spelt flour pita breads
- 4 ounces vegan mozzarella, shredded
- 1 cup mixed veggies of your choice (tomatoes, eggplant, onion, green pepper, mushroom, etc.), rinsed and finely sliced

- ⅔ cup pitted olives, chopped
- 1 tablespoon extra-virgin olive oil
- 5 fresh basil leaves, rinsed and torn

Directions:

1. For the Sauce
2. In a blender, blend the tomatoes, olive oil, basil, garlic, onion powder, oregano, sage, rosemary, chili flakes, salt, and pepper on low until the basil and garlic are in very small pieces.
3. Place it on a pot over medium heat and simmer for about 20 minutes, until the sauce reduces slightly and thickens.
4. For the Pizza
5. Line the baking sheet and preheat the oven to 500degrees then set aside.
6. Spread the pizza sauce evenly over the pitas. Top with the vegan mozzarella and scatter the sliced veggies and olives on top. Bake until golden on top.
7. Drizzle the pizzas with the olive oil and scatter the basil leaves over them. Freeze leftovers in an airtight container for up to three weeks.

Nutrition:

400 calories | 10g total fat | 64g total carbohydrates | 5g fiber | 10g protein

Tomato Spelt Pasta

Preparation Time: 15 minutes

Cooking Time: 20 minutes

Serving: 4

Ingredients

- 3 tablespoons extra-virgin olive oil
- 2 garlic cloves, crushed
- 1 onion, rinsed and diced
- 1 eggplant, rinsed and diced
- 2 zucchinis, rinsed and diced
- 3 tomatoes, rinsed and diced
- ⅔ cup sun-dried tomatoes
- 2 teaspoons dried basil
- 1 teaspoon dried oregano
- 1 cup vegetable stock
- 1 tablespoon red wine vinegar
- Himalayan pink salt
- Freshly ground black pepper
- 7 ounces spelt pasta
- Boiling filtered water

Directions:

1. Heat olive oil over medium heat. Add the garlic, onion, and eggplant, and sauté for 8 minutes. Add the zucchini, tomatoes, sun-dried tomatoes, basil, and oregano. Cook for 8 minutes, stirring.

2. Stir in the vegetable stock and vinegar, and season with salt and pepper. Let simmer for a few minutes. In the meantime, in a different saucepan over medium heat, add in the pasta with enough boiling water to cover and cook for about 10 minutes, until soft. Drain.

3. Serve the pasta with the sauce.

Nutrition:

460calories | 12g total fat | 75g total carbohydrates | 10g fiber | 11g sugar | 17g protein

Tropical Mushrooms

Preparation Time: 20 minutes

Cooking Time: 10 minutes

Serving: 4

Ingredients

- ¼ cup coconut oil
- 2 portobello mushrooms, cleaned and sliced
- 2 onions, rinsed and sliced
- 1 green bell pepper, rinsed and sliced
- 2 garlic cloves, minced
- 1 cup chopped pineapple
- ¼ cup pure maple syrup or coconut palm sugar
- 2 tablespoons freshly squeezed lemon juice
- Himalayan pink salt
- Freshly ground black pepper

Directions:

1. Heat the coconut oil over medium heat. Add the mushrooms, onions, green pepper, and garlic. Cook for 5 to 7 minutes, until the vegetables are soft and turning golden brown.

2. Turn the heat to low. Stir in the pineapple, maple syrup, and lemon juice, and season with salt and

pepper. Simmer for 3 minutes to warm through, and serve.

Nutrition:

245 calories | 14g total fat | 30g total carbohydrates | 3g fiber | 22g sugar | 2g protein

Homemade Protein Bar

Preparation Time: 5 minutes

Cooking Time: 10 minutes

Servings: 4

Ingredients:

- 1 cup nut butter
- 4 tablespoons coconut oil
- 2 scoops vanilla protein
- Stevia, to taste
- ½ teaspoon sea salt
- Optional Ingredients:
- 1 teaspoon cinnamon

Directions:

1. Mix coconut oil with butter, protein, stevia, and salt in a dish. Stir in cinnamon and chocolate chip.
2. Press the mixture firmly and freeze until firm. Cut the crust into small bars. Serve and enjoy.

Nutrition:

179 Calories | 15.7g Total Fat | 4.8g Total Carbs | 3.6g Sugar | 0.8g Fiber | 5.6g Protein

Shortbread Cookies

Preparation Time: 10 minutes

Cooking Time: 70 minutes

Servings: 6

Ingredients:

- 2 1/2 cups almond flour
- 6 tablespoons nut butter
- 1/2 cup erythritol
- 1 teaspoon vanilla essence

Directions:

1. Line the cookie sheet and preheat your oven to 350 degrees. Beat butter with erythritol until fluffy.
2. Stir in vanilla essence and almond flour. Mix well until crumbly. Spoon out a tablespoon of cookie dough onto the cookie sheet. Add more dough to make as many cookies. Bake for 15 minutes until brown. Serve.

Nutrition: 288 Calories | 25.3g Total Fat | 9.6g Total Carbs | 3.8g Fiber | 76g Protein

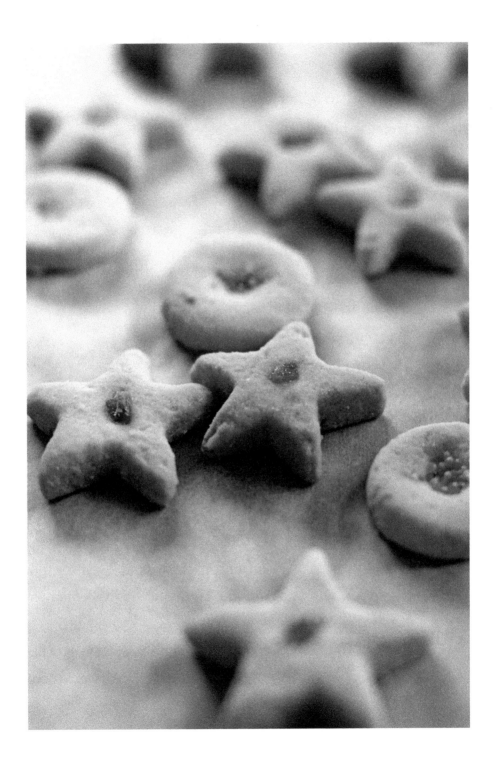

Coconut Cookies

Preparation Time: 10 minutes

Cooking Time: 15 minutes

Servings: 4

Ingredients:

- 1 cup almond flour
- ½ cup cacao nibs
- ½ cup coconut flakes, unsweetened
- 1/3 cup erythritol
- ½ cup almond butter
- ¼ cup nut butter, melted
- ¼ cup almond milk
- Stevia, to taste
- ¼ teaspoon sea salt

Directions:

1. Line the cookie sheet and preheat your oven to 350 degrees. Add and combine all the dry ingredients in a glass bowl.
2. Whisk in butter, almond milk, vanilla essence, stevia, and almond butter. Beat well then stir in dry mixture. Mix well.

3. Spoon out a tablespoon of cookie dough on the cookie sheet then add more dough to make as many as 16 cookies.

4. Flatten each cookie using your fingers and bake for 25 minutes until golden brown.

5. Let them sit for 15 minutes. Serve.

Nutrition:

192 Calories | 17.44g Total Fat | 2.2g Total Carbs | 1.4g Sugar | 2.1g Fiber | 47g Protein

Coconut Cookies

Preparation Time: 10 minutes

Cooking Time: 20 minutes

Servings: 6

Ingredients:

- 6 tablespoons coconut flour
- ¾ teaspoons baking powder
- 1/8 teaspoon sea salt
- 3 tablespoons nut butter
- 1/6 cup coconut oil
- 6 tablespoon swerves
- 1/3 cup coconut milk
- 1/2 teaspoon vanilla essence

Directions:

1. Line the cookie sheet and preheat your oven to 375 degrees. Beat all the wet ingredients in a mixer. Mix all the dry mixture in a blender. Stir in the wet mixture and mix well until smooth.
2. Spoon a tablespoon of cookie dough on the cookie sheet and add more dough to make as many cookies. Bake until golden brown. Serve.

Nutrition:

151 Calories | 13.4g Total Fat | 6.4g Total Carbs | 2.1g Sugar | 4.8g Fiber

Blueberry Mousse

Preparation Time: 10 minutes

Cooking Time: 25 minutes

Servings: 4

Ingredients:

- 1 teaspoon lemon zest
- 3 oz. raspberries or blueberries
- ¼ teaspoon vanilla essence
- 2 cups coconut cream

Directions:

1. Blend cream in an electric mixer until fluffy. Stir in vanilla and lemon zest. Mix well.
2. Fold in nuts and berries. Cover the bowl with a plastic wrap. Refrigerate for 3 hours. Garnish as desired. Serve.

Nutrition:

265 Calories | 13g Total Fat | 7.5g Total Carbs | 0.5g Fiber | 5.2g Protein

Almond Pulp Cookies

Preparation Time: 5 minutes

Cooking Time: 10 hours

Servings: 4

Ingredients:

- 3 cups almond pulp
- 1 Granny Smith apple
- 1-2 teaspoon cinnamon
- 2-3 tablespoons raw honey
- 1/4 cup coconut flakes

Directions:

1. Blend almond pulp with remaining ingredients in a food processor. Make small cookies out this mixture. Place them on a cookie sheet, lined with parchment paper. Place the sheet in a food dehydrator for 6 to 10 hours at 115 degrees F. Serve.

Nutrition:

240 Calories | 22.5g Total Fat | 17.3g Total Carbs | 14.9g Protein

Coconut Raisins cookies

Preparation Time: 10 minutes

Cooking Time: 10 minutes

Servings: 4

Ingredients:

- 1 1/4 cup almond flour
- 1 cup coconut flour
- 1 teaspoon baking soda
- 1/2 teaspoon Celtic sea salt
- 1 cup nut butter
- 1 cup coconut palm sugar
- 2 teaspoons vanilla
- ¼ cup almond milk
- 3/4 cup organic raisins
- 3/4 cup coconut chips or flakes

Directions:

1. Set your oven to 357 degrees F. Mix flour with salt and baking soda. Blend butter with sugar until creamy then stirs in almond milk and vanilla. Mix well then stir in dry mixture. Mix until smooth.
2. Fold in all the remaining ingredients. Make small cookies out this dough. Arrange the cookies on a

baking sheet. Bake for 10 minutes until golden brown.

Nutrition:

237 Calories | 19.8g Total Fat | 55.1g Total Carbs | 0.9g Fiber

Greek Zucchini Cups

Preparation Time: 10 minutes

Cooking Time: 5 minutes

Servings: 2

Ingredients

- 2 medium zucchinis, cut into 2-inch pieces and each piece slightly cored to form a cup
- 1 cucumber, finely grated
- 1 cup plain Greek yogurt
- 1 garlic clove, minced
- 1 tablespoon dill, chopped
- 1 tablespoon parsley, chopped
- 1 tablespoon lemon juice
- ½ teaspoon Himalayan salt
- ½ teaspoon black pepper, crushed
- 10 black olives, finely chopped
- 2 tablespoons sprouts

Directions:

1. Prepare zucchini cups and set aside. In a bowl, mix together cucumber, yogurt, garlic, dill, parsley, lemon juice, salt and pepper. Spoon into zucchini cups. Top each cup with some of the olives and sprouts.

Nutrition:

148 calories | 14g sugar | 35g protein

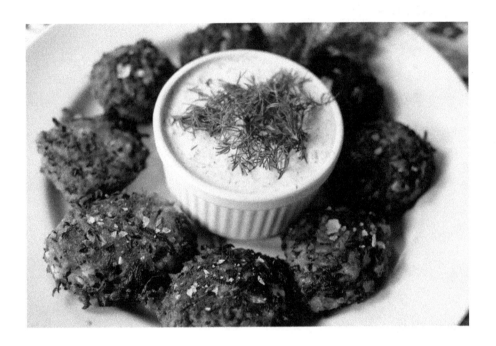

Endive & Watercress Boats

Preparation Time: 5 minutes

Cooking Time: 15 minutes

Servings: 2

Ingredients

- 3 cups fresh spinach
- 1 avocado
- 1/2 cup parsley
- ¼ cup mint
- 1 tablespoon lemon juice
- 1 garlic clove
- 1 teaspoon Himalayan salt
- 10 endive leaves
- 1 cup watercress

Directions:

1. Add all ingredients expect the endive leaves & watercress to a blender or food processor and blend until smooth, this will form the dip.
2. Scoop dip into each of the endive leaves and top with watercress.

Nutrition:

204 Calories | 17g Fiber | 29g Protein

Toasted Trail Mix

Preparation Time: 5 minutes

Cooking Time: 10 minutes

Servings: 2

Ingredients

- 3 tablespoons coconut chips, toasted
- 3 tablespoons walnuts, toasted
- 2 tablespoons almonds, toasted
- 2 tablespoons raisins
- 1 tablespoon pepitas, toasted
- Pinch Himalayan salt

Directions:

1. Combine all ingredients and divide into two equal portions

Nutrition:

200 calories | 28g fiber | 39g protein

Chickpea Avocado Cups

Preparation Time: 20 minutes

Cooking Time: 5 minutes

Servings: 1

Ingredients

- 1 very ripe avocado
- ½ cup cooked chickpeas
- ½ tomato, diced
- 1 shallot, diced
- 2 tablespoons olive oil
- 1 tablespoon lemon juice
- ½ teaspoon Himalayan salt
- ½ teaspoon black pepper, crushed
- 1 tablespoon fresh basil, chopped
- 1 teaspoon oregano

Directions:

1. In a small bowl combine chickpeas, tomato, shallot, olive oil, lemon juice, salt and black pepper. Set aside and let rest 5 minutes.

2. Slice the avocado in half lengthwise and remove the pit. Spoon the chickpea and tomato mixture over the

middle of each avocado. Garnish with oregano and fresh basil.

Nutrition:

150 calories | 14g fiber | 28g protein

Spicy Cocoa-Coco Truffles

Preparation Time: 10 minutes

Cooking Time: 20 minutes

Servings: 2

Ingredients

- 2 cups pitted dates
- ½ cup almond meal
- 1/3 cup shredded unsweetened coconut
- 6 tablespoons raw cacao (or unsweetened cocoa) powder, divided
- ¼ teaspoon sea salt
- ¼ teaspoon cayenne pepper

Directions:

1. Using a food processor on the pulse setting combine the dates, almond meal and shredded coconut until crumbly.
2. Add in 3 tablespoons of the cacao, the sea salt and the cayenne. Blend until the mixture becomes a sticky paste and begins to form a ball.
3. Shape the dough into 6 balls. Place remaining cacao on a plate and roll each ball lightly in the cacao.

Nutrition:

139 calories | 25g fiber | 40g protein | 11g sugar

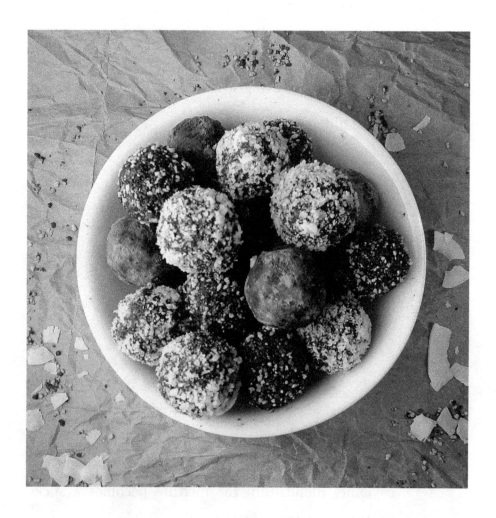

Toasty Quinoa

Preparation Time: 5 minutes

Cooking Time: 25 minutes

Serving: 2

Ingredients:

- 3 cups coconut milk
- 1 cup quinoa, rinsed
- 1/8 teaspoon ground cinnamon
- 1 cup raspberry
- ½ cup chopped coconuts

Directions:

1. Add milk into a saucepan and bring to a boil over high heat. Add quinoa to the milk and again bring it to a boil. Let it simmer for 15 minutes, on low heat until milk is reduced. Stir in cinnamon and mix well.

2. Cover and cook for 8 minutes until milk is completely absorbed. Add raspberry and cook for 30 seconds. Serve and enjoy.

Nutrition:

271 Calories | 3.7g Fat | 54g Carbs | 6.5g Protein | 3.5g Fiber

Tropical Pancakes

Preparation Time: 5 minutes

Cooking Time: 15 minutes

Serving: 4

Ingredients:

- 1 cup coconut flour
- 2 tablespoons arrowroot powder
- teaspoon baking powder
- 1 cup coconut milk
- 3 tablespoons coconut oil

Directions:

1. Mix all dry ingredients in a medium container. Add coconut milk and 2 tablespoons coconut oil. Mix well. Melt a teaspoon coconut oil in a skillet.
2. Pour a ladle of the batter into the skillet and swirl the pan to spread it into a smooth pancake. Cook for 3 minutes on low heat until firm then continue cooking both sides until golden brown. Cook more pancakes using the remaining batter. Serve.

Nutrition:

377 Calories | 14.9g Fat | 60.7g Carbs | 6.4g Protein | 1.4g Fiber

Quinoa Grout

Preparation Time: 5 minutes

Cooking Time: 25 minutes

Serving: 2

Ingredients:

- 2 cups coconut milk
- 1 cup quinoa, rinsed
- 1/8 teaspoon ground cinnamon
- 1 cup (1/2 pint) fresh blueberries

Directions:

1. Boil coconut milk in a saucepan over high heat. Add quinoa to the milk and again bring it to a boil. Let it simmer for 15 minutes on low heat until milk is reduced. Stir in cinnamon and mix well. Cover and cook for 8 mins until milk is completely absorbed. Add blueberries and cook for 30 seconds. Serve and enjoy.

Nutrition:

271 Calories | 3.7g Fat | 54g Carbs | 6.5g Protein | 3.5g Fiber

Amaranth Grout

Preparation Time: 5 minutes

Cooking Time: 30 minutes

Servings: 2

Ingredients:

- 2 cups coconut milk
- 2 cups alkaline water
- 1 cup amaranth
- 2 tablespoons coconut oil
- 1 tablespoon ground cinnamon

Directions:

1. Mix milk with water in a medium saucepan. Bring the mixture to a boil. Stir in amaranth then reduce the heat to low. Cook on low simmer for 30 minutes with occasional stirring.
2. Turn off the heat. Stir in cinnamon and coconut oil. Serve warm.

Nutrition:

434 Calories | 35g Fat | 27g Carbs | 6.7g Protein | 3.6g Fiber

Banana Barley Porridge

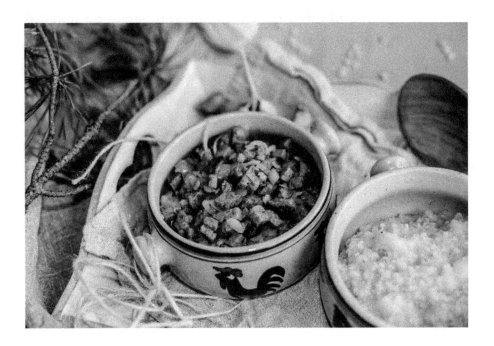

Preparation Time: 15 minutes

Cooking Time: 5 minutes

Servings: 2

Ingredients:

- 1 cup unsweetened coconut milk, divided
- 1 small banana, peeled and sliced
- ½ cup barley
- 3 drops liquid stevia
- ¼ cup coconuts, chopped

Directions:

1. Mix barley with half coconut milk and stevia in a bowl and mix well. Cover and refrigerate for about 6 hours. Mix the barley mixture with coconut milk in a saucepan. Cook for 5 minutes on medium heat. Top with chopped coconuts and banana slices. Serve.

Nutrition:

159 Calories | 8.4g Fat | 19.8g Carbs | 4.6g Protein | 4.1g Fiber

30 DAY MEAL PLAN

Day	Breakfast	Main Dishes	Snacks
1	Blackberry Pie	Kamut Burger	Avocado Basil Pasta
2	Blueberry Spelt Breakfast Muffins	Veggie Burgers	Rice and Spinach Balls
3	Alkaline Blueberry Breakfast Cake	Falafel with Tzatziki Sauce	Flatbread
4	Teff Sausages	Veggie Kabobs	Enoki Mushroom Pasta
5	Alkaline Breakfast Biscuits	Mushroom Curry	Walnut Kale Pasta
6	Zucchini Bacon	Veggies Casserole	Tomato Pasta
7	Alkaline Spelt Bread	Sweet and Spicy Chickpeas	Zucchini Tomato Pasta
8	Alkaline Crustless Quiche	Chickpea and Veggies Stew	Zucchini Bacon
9	Alkaline's Home Fries Hash Browns	Alkaline Pizza Crust	Alkaline Sausage Links
10	Alkaline Blueberry and Strawberry Muffins	Vegan Alkaline Ribs	Garlicky Broccoli

11	Teff Breakfast Porridge	Grilled Zucchini Hummus Wrap	Sautéed Kale
12	Alkaline Sausage Links	Veggie Fajitas Tacos	Parsley Mushrooms
13	Breakfast Blueberry Bars	Chickpea Mashed Potatoes	Speltbread
14	Alkaline Veggie Omelet	Wild Rice and Black Lentil Bowl	Tortillas
15	Butternut Squash Hash Browns	Cauliflower Alfredo Pasta	Tortilla Chips
16	Blueberry Spelt Flat Cakes	Zucchini Noodles with Avocado Sauce	Onion Rings
17	Blueberry Pie	Chinese Cucumber Salad Magnifico	Basil and Olive Pizza
18	Blueberry Spelt Breakfast Muffins	Artichoke Sauce Ala Quinoa Pasta	Tomato Spelt Pasta
19	Alkaline Blueberry Breakfast Cake	Beautifully Curried Eggplant	Tropical Mushrooms
20	Teff Sausages	Coconut Milk and Glazing Stir Fried Tofu	Shortbread Cookies
21	Alkaline Breakfast Biscuits	Culturally Diverse Pumpkin Potato Patties	Coconut Cookies

22	Zucchini Bacon	Italian Leek Fry	Blueberry Mousse
23	Alkaline Spelt Bread	Almond and Celery Mix of Delight	Almond Pulp Cookies
24	Alkaline Crustless Quiche	Spicy Tofu Burger	Toasted Trail Mix
25	Alkaline's Home Fries Hash Browns	Special Pasta Ala Pepper and Tomato Sauce	Chickpea Avocado Cups
26	Alkaline Blueberry and Strawberry Muffins	Southern Amazing Salad	Toasty Quinoa
27	Teff Breakfast Porridge	Pad Thai	Tropical Pancakes
28	Alkaline Sausage Links	Yellow Squash and Bell Pepper Bake	Quinoa Grout
29	Breakfast Blueberry Bars	Bell Peppers and Tomato Casserole	Squash Hash
30	Alkaline Veggie Omelet	Nori-Burritos	Blackberry Pie

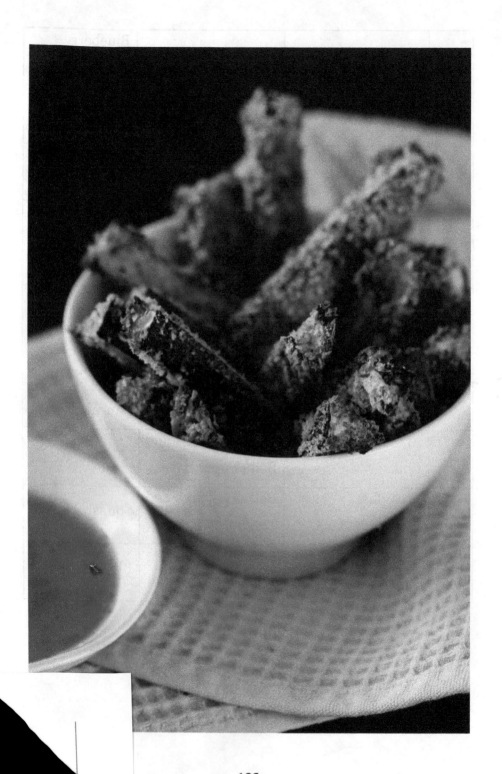